Digest Alive The Natural Cure to Heartburn

Written by Acharya D Hargreaves

Published 2007 by Lulu.com
Printed in the United States of America

ISBN 978-1-4303-1614-5

This is a reference work.
It is not meant for diagnosis or treatment and it is not a
substitute for consultation with a licensed health care provider.

Cover art designed by Acharya D Hargreaves

2

Digest Alive The Natural Cure to Heartburn

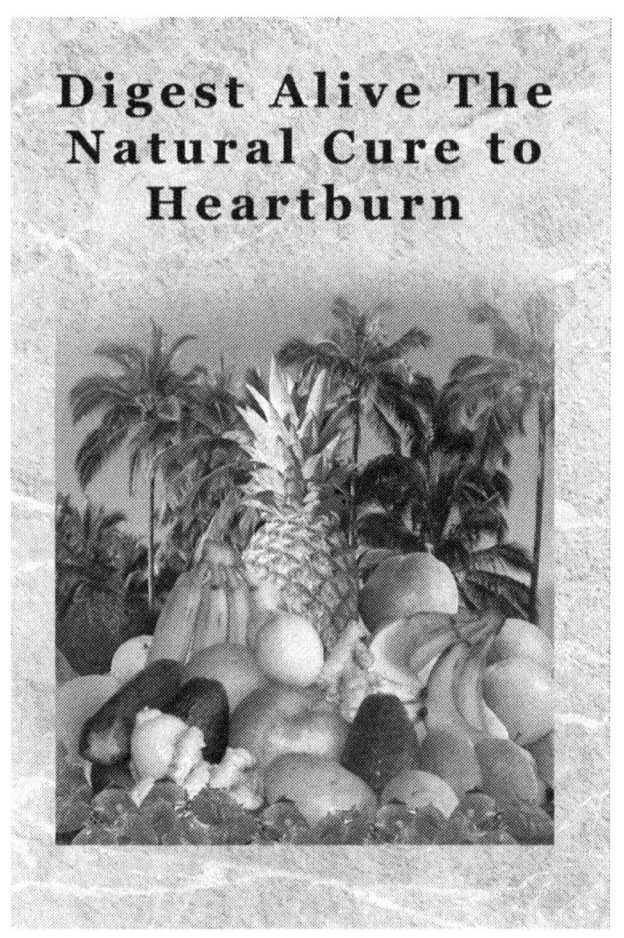

Digestion is the key

Life is not for surviving but for living

Acknowledgements

I would like to say thank-you to my wonderful family who have inspired me in my many goals and desires to succeed in my life and who gave me inspiration in writing this small book.

I also want to give special thanks to Harikirtana das, my brother, who gave me the idea of writing down how I cured my conditions, so others could benefit.

I sincerely hope and desire that anyone who reads this book will get help from some of my suggestions in curing their Heartburn, Acid reflux, Indigestion, Bad breath or any other digestive problem they may have.

Table of Contents

10

Introduction

Hello my name is Acharya D Hargreaves. I am the author of *Digest Alive The Natural Cure to Heartburn*

I once had a terrible case of heartburn and acid reflux. Through sheer desperation, I learned how to cure myself.

When I had the condition, I could not eat anything without getting a burning feeling inside me. So, I went to the doctors to see what they could do for me. The doctor put me on an antacid pill, but it only made things worse.

The antacid pill only stopped my pain for a very short while and than it was back even more powerfully then before. I started to feel sluggish and tired everyday and had more bad gas than usual. I also started having headaches and diarrhea.

I began to realize that these were possible side effects of the antacid drug I was taking. So I did a computer search and found that there were hundreds of possible side effects. I was actually harming my body instead of helping it. I decided then to stop taking the drug. When I stopped my body went into much greater pain than ever before.

Things were getting out of hand, so I became determined to fight my heartburn pains! My doctor could not help me and no one else could tell me what to do. I had to heal myself. That was the only option.

I knew the answers were out there somewhere. I became completely dedicated to finding a natural cure to my condition. I wanted to find a natural treatment as opposed to drugs.

It took me months of hard research to find a natural cure. I did extensive research on the use of herbs, home remedies, diets, aromatherapy, exercise, meditation, Asian medicine and much more. By trial and error, I finally discovered how I could cure these digestive disorders, which had given me pain for so long.

What I found out helped me immensely. In only six weeks of following a simple routine, my stomach stopped giving me gas after I ate and I hardly ever get Acid reflux or heartburn any more. I also found out that it helped my bad breath disappear. It was amazing.

I have been following this simple routine everyday now and I feel healthier than ever before. To me, health is wealth! Feeling healthy is number one in my book.

Chapter One
What creates heartburn?

Did you know that because of our rich diets and lifestyles, most of the time we will put large amounts of abuse on our digestive systems? Many of us eat too fast, or we swallow our food down followed by a very cold drink of some kind.

Unfortunately, our bodies have ways of getting back at us. They provide us with upset stomachs, burping, diarrhea and other digestive tract disorders.

A lot of the time we eat either too much, too little, too often or not often enough, we eat too quickly, while on the move or before bed? In addition, sometimes we simply eat foods that do not agree with us. Sometimes even our emotions have affects on how well we digest our food. If you or I are upset and we eat a big meal, usually we will suffer afterwards.

Having a properly working digestion is essential for a long and healthy life. Food you eat goes down the esophagus and through a valve into the stomach. Once in the stomach the food is further broken down by stomach acids and digestive enzymes secreted by digestive glands in the stomach lining these digestive enzymes help digest proteins.
After the digestive enzymes properly digest the food, it then moves into the intestines, which

starts absorbing the food, the waste is evacuated from the body.

If you are not absorbing or digesting your food properly, then problems can arise at any point in this process. Indigestion can ruin not just a meal but your whole day.

The foods you eat affect the air you breath out

Here is an interesting fact. According to the American Dental Association (ADA) "The foods you eat affect the air you exhale."

Once the food is digested and absorbed into the bloodstream, the nutrients are transferred all over the body including the lungs, where they are breathed out. That is why when you eat garlic or onion your breath smells like that for sometime, until your body has properly digested everything.

Brushing, flossing and mouthwash as well as many other types of fresheners will only make the odor temporarily disappear. The odor will continue until the body utilizes the food.

Not brushing or flossing daily can lead to particles of food that remain in the mouth. The bacteria grows on the food, which can cause bad breath. The food particles that collect between the teeth, on the tongue and around the gums can rot, leaving an unpleasant odor.

The ADA also says, Bad breath can also be caused by dry mouth also known as (xerostomia), which occurs when the flow of saliva decreases. Saliva is necessary to cleanse the mouth and remove particles that may cause odor.

What happens in the human body?

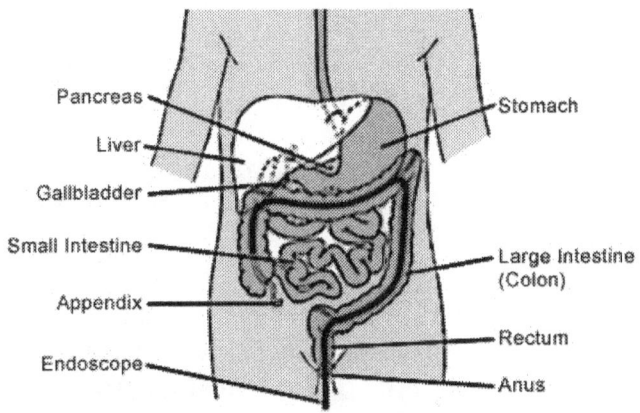

Now let's get down to business. Improperly digested food or undigested waste materials in the body are the root cause of Acid reflux, Heartburn, Indigestion and Bad breath.

Stomach acid is hydrochloric acid. Not enough stomach acid to properly digest the food, is the start of heartburn. When the body is trying to digest food and does not have enough of the acid, digestive enzymes or the acid is too weak to properly digest everything, the food that is only partially digested starts to ferment, causing gas and other problems in the system.

Poorly digested food becomes toxic when it sits too long in the upper stomach. As it sits, it can be absorbed into the body, causing stress for the liver and the immune system, eventually causing disease. If the body works too hard to digest food, vital energy is used and the body becomes weak.

Digestion starts in the mouth. When you chew your food, you break it into tiny parts so that your stomach can break down the food further.

Cathy Wong, a licensed naturopathic doctor, states in her article "chewing is the best way to help your digestion".

Chewing is one of the best ways to help your digestion in its process, because when you chew your food well, your saliva starts to digests your food first in your mouth before it even reaches your stomach. This process is the most important in helping your digestion to assimilate your food.

The saliva glands are the first to act on digesting what you eat. When you chew your food, your saliva mixes with it and starts a chemical digestion of the food particles.

Your saliva stimulates the exocrine glands in the mouth to release digestive enzymes into the food that start a chemical breakdown of it, particularly carbohydrates. Then, your stomach will not work so hard.

After the food enters your stomach, your food gets further broken down through a process of heuristic churning and is then mixed with a digestive fluid that is made up of hydrochloric acid and other digestive enzymes. This digestive fluid helps to further breakdown proteins.

If your system does not have enough hydrochloric acid or digestive enzymes, then your stomach will have a hard time properly digesting all the food and the food will start to become toxic. This is the start of bloating, feeling acidy and burpy, gas and bad breath.

What is acid reflux?

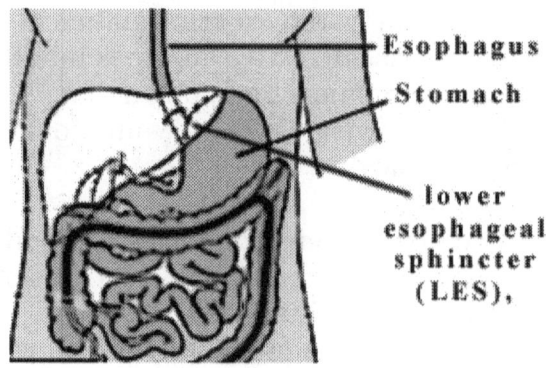

Esophagus

Stomach

lower
esophageal
sphincter
(LES),

Most people believe that, too much acid causes acid reflux and heartburn. Actually, this is not the case.

According to Dr. Elena Koles, MD, "heartburn and acid reflux are caused by a lack of stomach acid".

Acid reflux takes place because of blockage in the stomach. Hydrochloric acid is forced upwards towards, the esophagus by a build up of fermentation gas.

If there is not enough hydrochloric acid or digestive enzymes to digest everything properly, the food starts to ferment. The fermentation of undigested foods produces large amounts of gas that push stomach acid

18

and food back up the esophagus.

Bad digestion and overeating can weaken the lower esophageal sphincter or (LES). At the top of your stomach or the bottom of your esophagus is a muscle called the lower esophageal sphincter (LES), which lets food in by opening and shutting. In addition, it shields the esophagus by blocking stomach acid from going up.

The LES is responsible for closing and opening the lower end of the esophagus and is essential for maintaining a pressure barrier against hydrochloric acid. The LES is a complex area of muscles and various hormones. If the LES weakens, then it cannot close up completely after food empties into the stomach.

The acid from the stomach is pushed up into the esophagus by the fermenting gas and the feeling associated with this is usually heartburn or acid reflux. The fermentation of undigested food also produces a sour gassy vapor that causes a sour stomach and bad breath.

Heartburn is a pain or burning sensation right behind the breastbone. Many people suffer from heartburn but heartburn has nothing to do with the heart. Heartburn is a digestive problem and is usually caused by meals and posture.

When someone feels heartburn, it is because their digestion is not putting out enough hydrochloric acid or digestive enzymes to digest the food properly or the hydrochloric acid is too weak to digest everything.

The food that is not fully digested starts to ferment and the gas produced causes the rise of hydrochloric acid up through the LES. When the stomach acid touches the lining of the esophagus, it causes a burning sensation in the chest or throat. That is called heartburn.

According to some health professionals, the long-term use of antacids or acid blockers can lead to even more complex and long-term health risks including poor absorption increased risk of intestinal infections and tumors of the stomach.

How you can cure your heartburn and indigestion

Ok. Here are the steps you should take if you want to cure your stomach problems. These steps should be performed everyday. If you do not follow these steps everyday and keep a routine going, then your digestion will not get the help it needs to become stronger.

First off, remember to chew your food until it is almost liquid. That will greatly help in your digestion, since your saliva will have adequately performed its digestion process. It may not sound so appealing but this simple task will improve things immensely.

Remember not to eat too much. Overeating will cause fermentation and gas to start to build up inside your stomach.

Your stomach only has a certain amount of hydrochloric acid and digestive enzymes each time that you eat, so if you have too much food in your stomach, the food will not get digested properly and will start to ferment. So, eat only until you feel almost full and then stop.

A good way to measure is to eat only until you have your first or second burp. Your body is telling you something. Listen to it and stop when you burp.

According to some professionals, it is not advisable to eat during bedtime hours, because your stomach stops working then. Around 8:00 or 9:00 PM, your stomach stops performing its digestion and your body starts getting everything ready for resting and recovery for the next day.

If you do eat food during bedtime hours what happens is the food sits in your stomach, overnight and ferments, causing damage to your digestive enzymes for the next day and can give you bad breath in the morning.

Eating on a regular timetable or schedule helps

as well. It will help to maintain a balanced digestion.

The digestion in our body is like the element of fire and one of the best ways to intensify a fire is to feed it oxygen. Therefore, if you can do some exercise before you eat then your digestion will improve and your body will be able to digest the food better.

Jogging, swimming, walking all do the job. Exercise builds appetite and a well-oxygenated body creates higher temperatures, which then helps to achieve combustion that is more efficient.

If you do not want to do exercise before you eat, then do 5 minutes of deep breathing just before your meal. This will help to increase digestion for proper assimilation.

Also relaxing while you eat is a great way to help your digestion in its process. Sit down in a comfortable place and enjoy your food as much as possible. That way, your body is not under any kind of stress and can accept the food that is put into it more easily.

Stress is also a very big cause of heartburn and acid reflux. If you are stressed out when you have acid reflux or heartburn try to relax and take a few deep breaths.

One of the best ways of reducing stress is to breath deep three times and then ask your mind a positive question that has nothing to do with what you were thinking about.

Physiologists say that the brain can only think of one thing at a time and if you can remove the painful or negative thought with a more positive thought then your pain or stress will instantly go away.

Try to think positively while you are eating. Thinking positively all day, actually, is great. However, it takes sometime to get used to thinking this way.

Also listening to soothing music that calms your nerves and relaxes you is an excellent way to feel more relaxed when eating. I personally like to listen to Indian classical music while I am eating.

Ok. So, here we go.

Number One: You chew your food until it is almost liquid.

Number Two: Remember not to eat too much. Use your first or second burp as a guideline.

Number Three: No eating during bedtime hours. The stomach stops performing its digestion at this time and your body starts getting everything ready for resting and recovery for the next day.

Number Four: Relax for the best effect. Be in a

relaxed calm state for your digestion to have its best effect.

Yoga exercises to help improve your overall digestion

If you are interested in Yoga, then here are a few Yoga exercises that will help to improve your overall digestion. Practicing these poses daily on an empty stomach will help digestion.

You can find these yoga poses in many yoga books as well as many more poses that are beneficial to your health. Yoga exercise is a great way to help balance your whole body.

Caution: It is a good idea to avoid these poses if you have had a hiatal hernia or abdominal surgery, have abdominal inflammation, a hyperthyroid condition, diarrhea, sciatica, or back problems, or are pregnant or menstruating. If you still want to practice them ask your doctor if they are ok for you.

The cobra

1. #A Lie on your stomach with your forehead on the floor and your legs together. Also put your hands, palms down, under your shoulders.

2. #B When you inhale, bring your head up, brushing first your nose, then your chin against the floor. Now, push up with your hands and use your back muscles to raise your chest as high as possible. Hold this pose for a few deep breaths and then exhale slowly. Return to position 1. #A, keeping your chin up until last.

3. #C Then Inhale again and come up as before, but this time use your hands to push the trunk up. Continue up until you are bending from the middle of the spine. Hold this position for two or three deep breaths and then exhale and come slowly down.

4. #C Again inhale and raise the trunk as before, but this time continue up and back until you can feel you're back bending all the way down from the neck to the base of the spine. Breathe normally and hold this position for as long as you feel comfortable, then slowly come down and relax.

The cobra poses

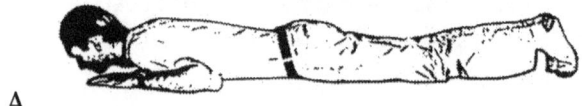

A

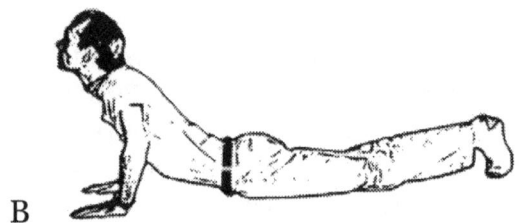

B

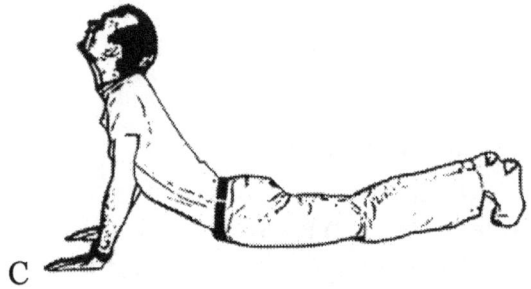

C

The bent elbow spinal twist

1. Sit on the floor with your legs extended out in front of you. Make sure your butt is firmly on the floor and that you maintain a straight spine or back. Do not round your back. Sitting on the edge of a cushion can prevent this.

2. #A Bend your right knee and plant your right foot on the floor near the inside of your left knee or thigh. Lift your left arm out in front of you, bend your elbow and place your elbow on the outside of your bent right knee with your palm facing away from you. Put your right hand on the floor behind you.

3. #B Now twist your torso to the right to look behind you and hold this position for 3 to 10 breaths. Each time you inhale, lengthen your spine to grow taller. Each time you exhale, twist to the right a little more.

4. Now, slowly turn back to the center and extend your legs out in front of you. Repeat this exercise on the opposite side.

The bent elbow poses

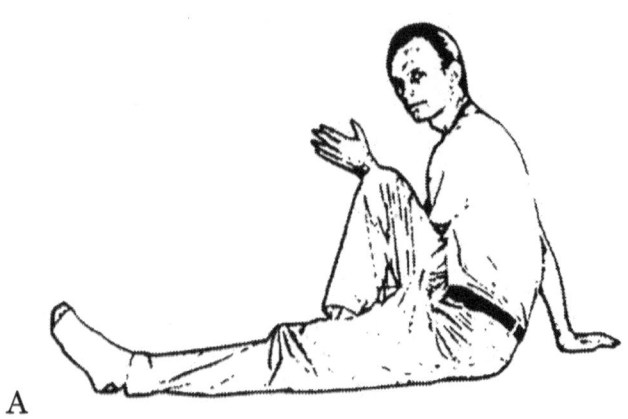

A

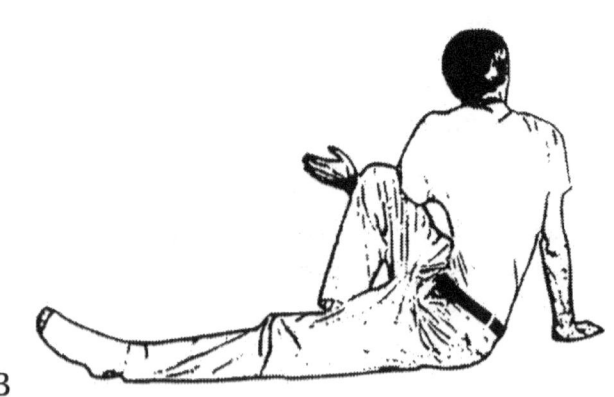

B

The hero

1. #A Sit on your butt with your knees bent and your feet flat on the floor, arms relaxed. Then slide your left foot under your right leg and next to your right hip. The outside of your left leg should be flat on the floor.

Next lift your right bent leg and cross it over your left knee, bringing your right foot as close to your left hip as you can. Move your right leg over only as far as feels comfortable.

To better position yourself, place your hands on the floor in front of you and lean forward, balancing on your knees. Then lower your buttocks to the floor.

2. #A Place your hands on the soles of your feet and lengthen your spine. Leading with your chest and folding from your hips, bend forward with a flat back. Stop every inch or so and breathe. You may not be able to come very far forward at first.

3. #B When you reach the point where you feel a stretch but not a strain, gently rest your chin on your chest. Hold this position for 3 to 10 breaths.

To release, press down into your buttocks and raise your torso with a straight strong back. Slowly unravel your legs using your hands to guide them back to the position in step 1.

Repeat for other side sliding your right leg under your left.

The hero poses

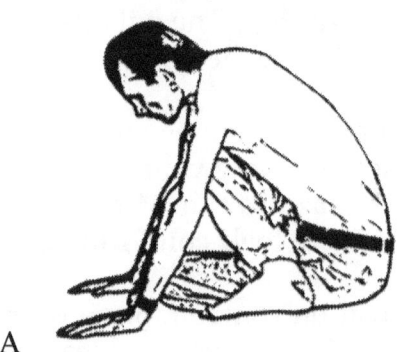

A

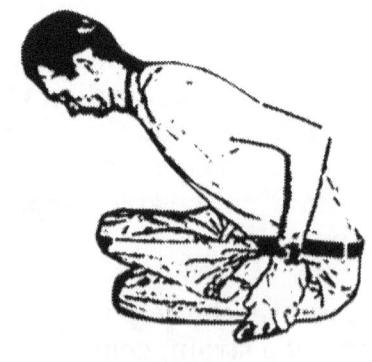

B

Different herbs to help your digestion

Here is a great list of before and after stomach helpers for your digestion, to help in the task of breaking down food into nutrients your body can properly absorb.

1. Lemon
Drinking a little lemon juice in hot water 20 minutes before a large protein meal will help your digestion in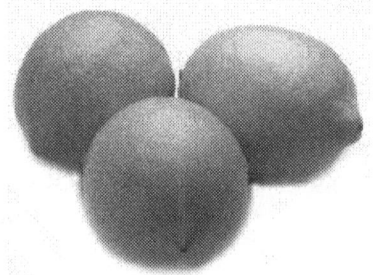
breaking down the food properly.
Lemon juice squirted on some foods like rice or in soups is good, also.

2. Bitters
Taking Swedish bitters daily will help with your digestion as well as other parts of your system. Bitter is strengthening.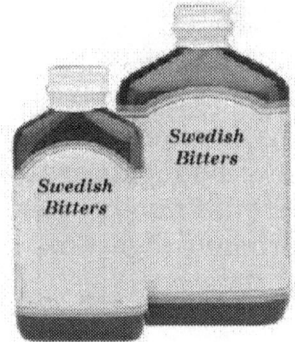

3. Fennel Taking a pinch full of Fennel seeds
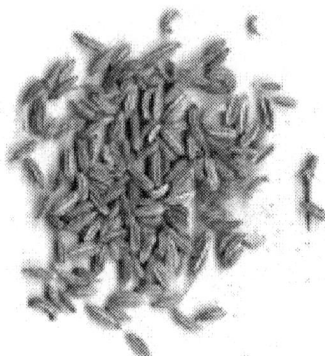
after every meal
helps the digestion
in its process of
assimilation. It helps
stomach gas and
gives a good smell to
your breath.

4. Peppermint is used primarily for treating
indigestion, flatulence (gas), and colic. It is
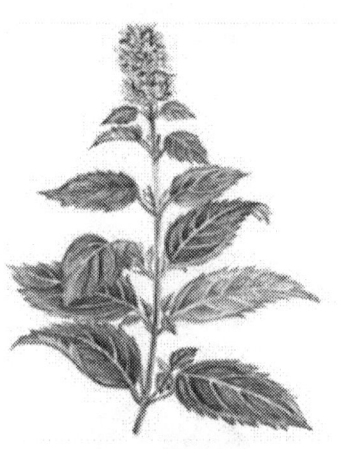
usually taken in a
warm tea prepared
from the leaves. One
cup slowly sipped
brings prompt relief.
Peppermint can also
be used as a pleasant
flavor for after eating.
American peppermint
oil contains from 50
to 78 percent of free
menthol and another
5 to 20 percent of
various combined forms (esters) of menthol.
These components are also responsible for
peppermint's ability to stimulate the bile flow
and promote digestion.

Digestive aids

You can also take a number of different types of digestive aids listed below, but before you decide on any one of the digestive aids it is a good idea to consult with a doctor.

A. Acidophilus is the friendly bacteria which lives in our intestine and keeps the harmful bacteria in check. If you use antibiotics, drugs, many times or drink chlorinated water and eat too many processed foods your bodies number of friendly bacteria in your intestine start to reduce. This paves the way for harmful bacteria to increase in number and cause disease.

Some people also have a intolerance to lactose, or dairy products. Acidophilus produces the enzyme lactase, which corrects this lactose intolerance problem. Acidophilus also produces B vitamins in the body, helps to cure bad breath, reduces cholesterol and also inhibits Candida albicans and prevents yeast infections.

33

B. Aloe Vera juice is rich in sulphur and 200 other nutrients. Aloe Vera juice aids the digestion and absorption of nutrients, helps control 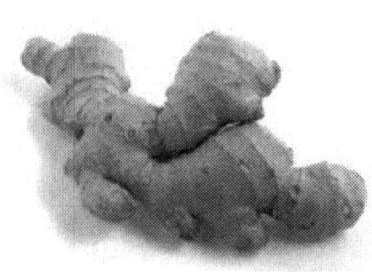 blood sugar, increases energy production, promotes cardiovascular health, improves liver function, and boosts the immune system.

C. Ginger aids in digestion from beginning to end. It is known as a sialagogue which promotes the secretion of saliva and thus, stimulates appetite. Ginger has been used for upset stomach and nausea. It aids in the digestion of proteins due to its high content of protease, an enzyme that helps break down proteins. The aromatic qualities of ginger also assist the digestive process.

Ginger stimulates the gastrointestinal mucous membranes, expels gas from the stomach and bowels. It increases the tone of the muscles and

34

stimulates peristalsis. It is often added to laxative formulas to prevent gripping.

D. Green Papaya Digestive Aid It is grown in the lava fields of Hawaii. Papaya is picked in a mature, green state because it is rich in two important enzymes that break down proteins, called Papain and Chymonpapain. The enzymes have a very powerful digestive action. The enzymes are stable in the 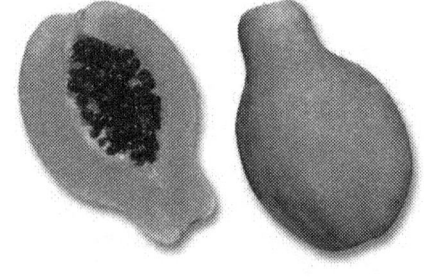 same range of acidity as the human gastric environment (1.0 to 1.8 pH).

These enzymes are most concentrated when the fruit is picked green. After a Papaya is picked, its enzymes start to dissipate as the fruit ripens and are not found at all in ripe papaya. Therefore, to offer the best concentrate and benefit of these enzymes, the papayas are picked green, cleaned, dried and processed before the fruit is allowed to ripen. Green Papaya taken regularly can also minimize the formation of ulcers in the human stomach.

E. Garlic is a very good food for the digestive system. Garlic exercises a beneficial effect on the lymph. It aids in the elimination of toxic 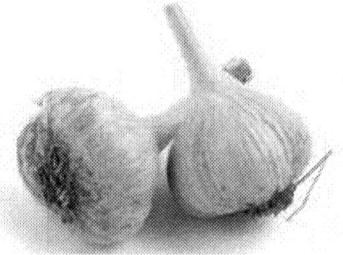 waste matter in the body. It stimulates peristaltic action and the secretion of the digestive juices.

Garlic is an excellent agent as a worm killer. And also has a soothing effect on different forms of diarrhea. In addition, problems such as colitis, dysentery and many other intestinal upsets can be successfully helped with fresh garlic or garlic capsules.

Garlic has the ability to destroy harmful bacteria in the intestines without affecting the beneficial organisms which aid digestion.

F. Parsley is great for odor absorbing and oxygenating chlorophyll. It is diuretic and is 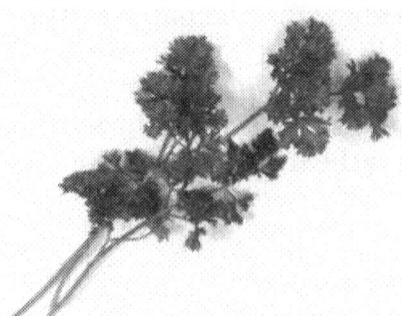 used in herbal formulas to build internal organs including kidney, thyroid, liver and prostate. Parsley is a

36

great digestive aid. It improves digestion and reduces cramping and gas after meals. Parsley also is a diuretic that helps get rid of excessive water. It provides plenty of potassium to balance the frequent excess of sodium in salt users.

G. Calcium is also very good for helping to overcome heartburn or acid reflux. Taking calcium everyday will increase the strength of your lower esophageal sphincter or LES, which lets food in by opening and shutting. When you strengthen this muscle you help prevent heartburn and acid reflux from ever happening again.

Best herbal teas to take for your digestion

Note: It is not recommended to make any tea with any sweeteners if you are trying to strengthen the immune system or ward off colds and flu. Sugars and sweeteners usually weaken the immune system.

Ginger tea is one of the best herbal teas for strengthening the digestion.

Hot ginger tea is an excellent winter drink. It will keep you warm and cozy. Use it to strengthen the digestion, improve circulation and ward off colds, sore throat and the flu.

Making Ginger tea is very simple

Recipe
Hot Water and fresh shredded ginger

Take 4 cups of water
a 2 inch piece of fresh ginger root
and if you want it sweet or tangy you can add honey and lemon

Peel the ginger root and slice it into thin slices. Bring the water to a boil in a saucepan. Once it is boiling, add the ginger. Cover the pot and reduce the heat to a simmer for 15-20 minutes. Strain the tea. Add honey and lemon for a sweet or tangy taste.

Chamomile Tea is great for digestive upset, flatulence, heartburn, muscle tension, diarrhea, anxiety and insomnia. Chamomile tea is also good for menstrual cramps, irritable bowel syndrome, tension headaches and restlessness.

Making chamomile tea is very simple

Recipe
Hot Water and dried chamomile

Take the dried chamomile and put one level teaspoon of the herb into a ceramic cup. After the water boils in a kettle or pot, pour hot water into the cup and cover for five minutes to let steep. You can drink the tea as it is or you can strain it into another cup. Use only ceramic, enamel or stainless steel pots or kettles when brewing the tea.

Peppermint Tea is a great blend to ease your stomach. Peppermint calms the muscles of the stomach and improves the flow of bile, which the body uses to digest fats. Food then passes through the stomach more quickly. Peppermint is a calming agent to soothe an upset stomach or to aid in digestion.

It has been used to treat headaches, skin irritations, anxiety associated with depression, nausea, diarrhea, menstrual cramps and flatulence. It is also widely used to treat symptoms of the common cold.

If your symptoms of indigestion are related to a condition called gastroesophageal reflux disease or GERD, peppermint should not be used.

Recipe
Hot Water and dried Peppermint leaves
Take a kettle or small pot and bring one cup of water to a boil, then turn off. Take the Peppermint leaves and put one half a tablespoon of the herb into the small pot or

kettle and let set for 5 to 10 minuets.

After the tea is finished, strain and drink it as it is or add sugar or honey for sweetener. Use only ceramic, enamel or stainless steel pots or kettles when brewing the tea. The tea can be made from leaves or dried leaves.

Other great digestive and health products

Online location to purchase these great items is listed at the top of each section.

Taken with permission from shokos.com

Herbal aloe force

http://www.shokos.com/Herbal-Aloe-Force-aloe-vera.htm

Herbal Aloe Force balances acid production, soothing and promoting optimal and original health of the entire gastrointestinal system.

Research has shown that aloe vera with its polysaccharides "re-natures" the cells of the body to function as they were originally

40

designed by nature.

Aloe with essiac's herbs fortifies cell walls strengthening cells resistance and integrity.

Cold processed Aloe Vera hydrates cells. It penetrates into cells 5 times more easily than water bringing in its own water and nutrients. (wetter than water!)

Cold processed Aloe Vera improves cellular metabolism - enhancing energy and optimal functioning of each cell of the body.

Cells eliminate toxins and waste more efficiently.

Aloe improves the efficient utilization of nutrients.

Digestion

Herbal Aloe Force's cold processed aloe vera with cat's claw, essiac's herbs, astragalus, pau d'arco, hawthorn berry and chamomile balances acid production, soothes and promotes optimal and original health of the entire gastrointestinal system for better absorption of nutrients along with improved elimination and detoxification.

Grifron maitake mushrooms

Maitake mushroom has a high content of 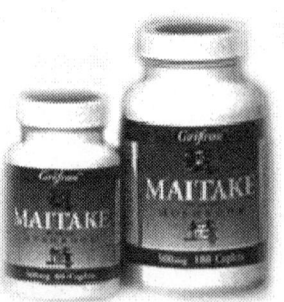 polysaccharide compound called beta glucan which stimulates the activities of immune cells. Maitake mushroom also contains valuable nutrients such as vitamin C, D, B2, niacin, minerals (especially magnesium, potassium and calcium), fiber and amino acids.

The whole maitake mushroom benefits as a tonic and is specifically useful in Weight loss, constipation, stimulating cellular immunity and is used during conventional cancer treatment to reduce cancers side effects such as hair loss, pain, fatigue and nausea. It also lowers blood pressure, reduces serum cholesterol, lowers blood sugar, uterine fibroids and inhibits tumor growth and metastasis.

Harmony colon formula colon cleansing

http://www.shokos.com/colonformula.htm

Harmony Colon Formula is a gentle, medium strength, yet effective colon cleanser that helps to jumpstart a sluggish and less efficient colon. Harmony Colon Formula is designed for individuals who experience approximately one bowel movement every 3 to 5 days.

Harmony Colon Formula addresses the deepest core of health! Our digestive system and colon keep us young, strong and energetic. It is where vital nutrients are extracted and absorbed from food, lending life and good health to our entire body.

Unfortunately, this system is also the most abused. We've been raised on a diet of bread, dairy, cheese, meat, fast foods, fried foods, fatty foods, sweets, candy, ice cream, etc. Over time, these foods can break down the digestive and eliminative system, making it function much less efficiently.

Bowel movements may slow to two to three times per week or less. Extremely sluggish or stubborn colons may need a gentle yet effective colon cleanser formula to get things moving again!

Digestive inefficiency can continue even after dietary improvements if you don't help rejuvenate your colon through internal colon cleansing. Harmony Colon Formula provides gentle strength for individuals who need it. Not all metabolisms are created equally. Some digestive and eliminative systems are simply more sluggish and less efficient. Stubborn may be the best way to describe them.

100% Pure, certified organic Tahitian noni juice

http://www.shokos.com/noni.html

Organic Tahitian Noni juice (morinda citrifolia) has been used by
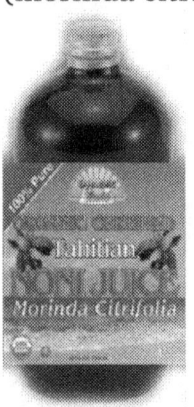
traditional Tahitian healers for thousands of years to improve general metabolism, strengthen the immune system, boost energy levels, improve circulation, promote healthy joints, support the digestive system, aid in the healing process, enhance overall vitality and impart a sense of well being.

This 100% Organic Tahitian

Noni juice contains a combination of unique substances, over 140 phytonutrients including selenium (a powerful anti-oxidant) and 3 important compounds: anthraquinones, damnacanthal and scopoletin.

It is believed that organic Noni juice works in the large intestine causing a chemical reaction that plays a key role in encouraging proper cell function and growth in the human body.
It enlarges the pores in the walls of human cells and enables nutrients to enter the cells more easily.

Extra virgin organic coconut oil

http://www.shokos.com/extra_virgin_coconut_oil.html

Botanical Medica's extra virgin organic coconut oil is rich in lauric acid, a prime ingredient in mothers' milk. Research has shown this to have anti-bacterial, anti-viral and anti-parasitic properties.

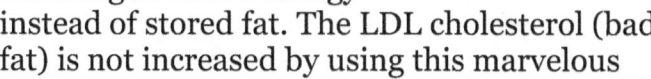

The medium chain fatty acids (MCFA's) are quickly metabolized by the body, resulting in added energy instead of stored fat. The LDL cholesterol (bad fat) is not increased by using this marvelous oil.

Nearly 50% of the fatty acid in extra virgin organic coconut oil is lauric acid, which converts to the fatty acid monolaurin in the body. Lauric acid has adverse effects on a variety of microorganisms including bacteria, yeast, fungi, and enveloped viruses. It destroys the lipid membrane of such enveloped viruses.

Extra virgin organic coconut oil provides an effective defense against many troublesome parasites including giardia. By using organic coconut oil and other coconut products everyday, you may be able to destroy giardia before it can establish a toehold. In so doing, you also eliminate the possibility of developing food allergies, fatigue and other related symptoms.

If you are currently troubled with these conditions, extra virgin organic coconut oil used liberally with meals may provide a source of relief. Another use for organic coconut oil is for the removal of intestinal worms. In India, it has been used to get rid of tapeworms naturally and is rubbed into the scalp as a natural treatment for head lice.

Chapter Two
The power of digestive enzymes

According to Ron Harder, a nutritional health consultant, "One of the most common health problems, today, is bad digestion"

One of the most common health problems today is bad digestion and the inability of our bodies to produce enough digestive enzymes and the lack of digestive enzymes in the food that we eat, both cause many problems that we have to face everyday.

What are digestive enzymes?

Digestive enzymes are molecules that break down food particles. When you chew, you break up the food into tiny bits. The digestive enzymes break the food particles into proteins, carbohydrates and fats. Then they are converted into smaller absorbable nutrients that your body can use to build cells, tissues and organs.

Digestive enzymes are responsible for breaking down the food into little tiny particles so that it can be more easily digested by the stomach and small intestine.

Digestion starts in the mouth. You put some food into your mouth and by chewing it, you break this food up into smaller pieces and mix it with saliva. Your saliva stimulates the exocrine glands in the mouth to release digestive enzymes into the food. That starts a chemical breakdown of the food.

When you chew your food, you break the food into tiny parts so your digestion can extract the nutrients. Chewing is one of the best ways to help your digestion in its process, because when you chew your food well your saliva starts digesting your food first in your mouth before it even reaches your stomach.

In the stomach your food is mixed with hydrochloric acid that helps to digest starches. More enzymes are added at this point which helps to break down your food even further and turn it into a paste-like substance called chyme.

After awhile, this chyme moves from the stomach to your small intestine where pancreatic enzymes are added to help with further digestion.

Where do digestive enzymes come from?

Ron Harder a nutritional health consultant, also states that "You obtain most of your digestive enzymes from the food that you eat."

Your body produces enzymes of its own and also, gets digestive enzymes from the food you eat. The body can only produce 16 digestive enzymes the other 8 digestive enzymes must be acquired from the food you eat.

Boiling and pasteurizing foods, destroy most of the enzymes that ever were in your food. Enzymes are also destroyed by temperatures over 118 degrees, cigarette smoke, caffeine, alcohol consumption and prescription drugs.

Plant enzymes are the best because they help begin digestion in your mouth. They are not destroyed by the acids in your stomach unlike animal enzymes and they function in both an acid and an alkaline environment. Animal enzymes can only live in an acid environment.

As we age, our body looses its ability to produce its own enzymes. So, we have to include them in our diet. You can get more enzymes by eating raw organic food and also by taking enzyme supplements.

Some good food sources for enzymes are

alfalfa, barley grass, chlorella, spirulina, kelp, peppermint and sea vegetables. Most fruits, especially bananas, are also a good source.

It is a good idea to make sure that you get enough enzymes, because a lack of digestive enzymes can cause a number of bodily problems.

Some of these problems can be heartburn, indigestion, constipation, abdominal bloating, colitis, diarrhea, eczema, IBD, psoriasis, skin rashes and many others.

Enzymes also help you to have a healthy balance of weight. If you do not have enough enzymes to properly digest all the food you eat, your body starts to store it as unwanted fats and other things. This is one of the causes of obesity.

If we have low levels of enzymes, the food becomes undigested and starts to ferment, causing our colon to become toxic. The toxic material that accumulates in our intestines will be absorbed through the intestinal wall and will end up in the blood stream.

Metabolic enzymes are responsible for the, repair and remodeling of every cell in our body. They are the workers within your body that allow the minerals, vitamins and proteins to do their job.

They are responsible for all the anabolic or

50

catabolic activity in your body. Metabolic enzymes are produced by the liver, pancreas and gallbladder.

Digestive enzymes in your diet

Taking enzyme supplements as part of your daily diet is a very good idea. It's quite easy and there are plenty of good enzyme supplements on the market today.

One I suggest is BioBuild. Taking enzyme supplements will ensure that you are getting all the enzymes that you need for your health.

Each enzyme can only do one specific job. One enzyme cannot do another enzymes job. So, if you are missing even just one enzyme it can have an impact on your health.

Enzymes are the first of the "workers" in your body. They are the catalysts that allow the minerals and vitamins in your body to do their job. They are responsible for all metabolic functions and most importantly they are responsible for life itself.

Here is a list of some of the main enzymes, their properties and what they help to achieve in your body.

If you would like to know more about each one of these enzymes you can look for more information on the web. There are many more enzymes than what I have listed here.

The digestive enzyme protease

This enzyme is responsible for digesting proteins in your food. Protease enzymes are found in the stomach, pancreatic, and intestinal juices. If the digestive process is incomplete, undigested protein can wind up in your circulatory system, as well as in other parts of your body. That's where this enzyme comes into play.

If you take the enzyme protease in higher quantities, your body takes the left over enzyme and uses it to help remove the unwanted protein from your circulatory system. This helps to clean up your blood stream and restore your energy and balance.

Protease also could help improve blood circulation, prevent abnormal blood clotting. Reduce pain and inflammation associated with Phlebitis, alleviate the pain, inflammation, and discomfort of varicose veins, minimize muscle

52

pain that occurs after exercise, minimize the inflammation and pain associated with Osteoarthritis and Rheumatoid Arthritis, alleviate the symptoms of Sinusitis and alleviate Edema.

Additional amounts of protease are also helpful in fighting such things as colds, flu's and cancerous tumor growths.

The enzyme Protease also helps in the healing and recovery from cancer. It dissolves the fibrin coating on cancer cells, and also gives your immune system a chance to do its job. This enzyme can effectively shrink the tumors by helping to remove the dead tissues, and by stimulating healthy tissue growth.

The digestive enzyme amylase

The second most important enzyme that we have is called Amylase. Amylase Enzymes, belonging to a family of alpha, beta and gamma digestive enzymes, are responsible for starch-splitting or amylolytic activity that splits starch molecules and related polysaccharides.

Amylase is responsible for digesting carbohydrates in food. Incomplete digestion of carbohydrates has been linked to blood sugar imbalances, allergies and asthma.

Amylase enzymes are also partly effective in destroying histamine reactions. Histamine reactions cause the general symptoms experienced during an allergic reaction, such as insect bites, pollen irritation, or contact with poison oak, poison ivy or poison sumac.

A possible reason why some people appear to be more immune to these poisons is because of a higher amount of amylase within their bodies.

The digestive enzyme lipase

This digestive enzyme is responsible for digesting fats in food. If taken in higher quantities it also helps to remove excess fat deposits from the inside of your veins and arteries through, the blood stream.

This enzyme is found in the stomach and pancreatic juice and is also found in fats from the foods that we eat. The Lipase enzyme helps to maintain a correct gall bladder function. The Lipase enzyme can also be helpful in weight loss, because it converts fat into energy instead of allowing it to be stored in your body.

The digestive enzyme cellulase

Cellulase is responsible for breaking down fiber. It is also an excellent antioxidant because it binds to heavy metals and other toxins and carries them out of your body. Cellulase digests cellulose fiber, and aids in malabsorption. The cellulase catalyzes the hydrolysis of cellulose fiber to cellobiose (a simpler cellulose chain). Present in intestinal bacteria.

We generally consume a combination of usable and unusable fiber. Usable fiber is effective in binding to excess cholesterol and toxic material and removing them from the body. Cellulase helps with this process, because it breaks down the usable fiber and allows it to be more efficient.

Unusable fiber provides the necessary bulk to keep the intestinal tract properly inflated and acts as a "push broom" to keep the walls of both the small and large intestines clean. Cellulase also helps to build and keep cells healthy.

The digestive enzyme lactase

This enzyme is responsible for digesting the milk sugar found in dairy products. Lactase is a common enzyme that exists in the small intestine of many people. It is essential for digestion of lactose, the naturally occurring sugar in milk.

However, not everyone produces enough lactase, resulting in difficulty or even inability to digest milk. Those who are "lactose intolerant" often suffer from symptoms including stomach cramps, gas and diarrhea.

The digestive enzyme maltase

The maltase enzyme takes the complex sugars found in grain products and changes it into glucose. When starch is eaten, it is partially digested and transformed into maltose by both the saliva enzymes and pancreatic enzymes. These enzymes are called amylases.

The maltase enzyme when secreted in the intestines, converts the maltose into a more usable sugar glucose.

The digestive enzyme phytase

The phytase enzyme helps with digestion in general and is especially effective in producing vital nutrients of the B-Complex. The phytase enzyme breaks down carbohydrates, specifically phytates or "phytic acid", which is present in many grains and beans that are difficult to digest.

This enzyme is useful for people suffering from serious bowel disorders which result in an inability to handle phytates from soy and gluten from wheat, oats, rye and barley. Phytase may increase mineral absorption and the bioavailability of iron, zinc, calcium and magnesium.

The digestive enzyme sucrase

This enzyme is responsible for digesting the sugars that are found in most foods. Sucrase is a yeast-derived enzyme. Sucrase splits sugar into glucose and fructose invert syrup.

Suggestions

Here are a few suggestions that you can follow to improve your overall health.

a) Chew your food well. This will help to break down your food so that your enzymes can do their job more effectively. This also will make the job your digestion has to do much easier and less stress on your system.

b) Eat your meals slowly. This will allow your food to proceed along your digestive tract in an orderly and continuous fashion. Enjoy your food as much as possible. When you are enjoying your food, your body is in a much happier state and can digest everything much easier.

c) Take time to relax after you eat so that your body will have the energy to start the digestive process.

d) Do not eat a heavy meal within three hours of bedtime, because your digestion is beginning to shut down for your resting time.

e) Drink plenty of water or herbal tea with and between your meals to promote better digestion and system regularity.

f) Eat plenty of fresh raw fruits and vegetables to maximize your enzyme intake.
Do your very best to obtain all the enzymes that you can. The more enzymes you consume, the

better your digestion will be and the more value you will obtain from your food. You don't have to worry about ever getting too many enzymes. They are not something on which you can overdose.

Make your own fruit juices, and smoothies

A great way to get more minerals and vitamins into your diet is by drinking freshly made fruit and vegetable juices.

Raw foods are rich in enzymes. Enzymes are needed for the digestive system to work. They are necessary to break down food particles so they can be utilized for energy. The human body makes approximately 22 different digestive enzymes which are capable of digesting carbohydrates, protein and fats. Raw vegetables and raw fruit are rich sources of enzymes.

The most powerful enzyme rich foods are sprouted seeds, grains and legumes. Sprouting increases the enzyme content in these foods a great deal.

Enzymes act as catalysts in hundreds of thousands of chemical reactions that take place throughout your body. They are essential for digesting, absorbing and converting food into body tissue.

Enzymes produce energy at the cellular level and are critical for most of the metabolic activities taking place in your body.

Drinking fresh juices and smoothies is one of the best ways your body can absorb more of the vitamins and minerals. If you eat the fruits and vegetables whole you do not get all the vitamins and enzymes out of the fruits or vegetables. Many of the nutrients are trapped in the fiber and by blending fruits and vegetables, you break down the fiber and release the vital nutrients.

Recipes to make homemade fruit and vegetable juices

Here is a small list for what you will need to make some fruit juices.

1. You will need a juice machine or blender. Either will do.

2. All the fruits and vegetables should be juiced raw to obtain the best amount of enzymes and

minerals. Cooked fruits or vegetables lose their digestive enzymes.

3. Organically grown fruits and vegetables are the best to juice because they do not contain any toxic chemical residue on their skins, but if you do use non organic fruit remember to peel it before juicing.

4. When juicing remember to remove the large pits from fruits like peaches, mangos, nectarines, etc.

5. It is always easier to juice cutup fruit. So, when you are ready to juice, cut all your fruit into small pieces that will fit easily into your blender or juicer.

6. When juicing do your best to juice fresh fruits and vegetables. The fresher they are the better. Under ripe fruits or vegetables will not juice well.

Homemade fruit juice recipes

Lemon lime ginger ale

Handful of grapes
1 apple, cored and sliced
½ inch fresh ginger (less if you find the taste too strong)
Juice of 1/2 lime
Juice of 1/4 lemon
sparkling mineral water

Remove the grapes from the stem. Juice the apple and ginger together, then add the rest of the juice. Pour the juice in a large glass, fill to the top with sparkling water and serve with ice.

Sparkling tropical fruit juice

1 kiwi, peeled
1 orange, peeled and sectioned
1/2 mango, peeled and sliced
sparkling mineral water

Process the fruit in a juicer or blender. Pour the juice in a large glass, fill to the top with sparkling water and serve.

Gingered apple cider juice

1 inch piece ginger
3 apples or 1 cup apple cider

Process through a juicer or blender and serve.

Peach pear apple juice

1 apple, cored and sliced
2 peaches, remove seed
1 pear, sliced

Process through a juicer or blender and serve.

Fruit punch juice

6 strawberries, fresh or thawed from frozen
1 apple, cored and sliced
1/2 orange, peeled and sectioned

Process the fruit in a juicer or blender and
serve.

Fruit nectar recipe

1/2 cup raspberries, fresh or thawed from frozen
1 orange, peeled and sectioned
1 nectarine, pitted and sliced

Process the fruit in a juicer or blender and serve.

Blueberry cherry juice recipe

Handful of cherries, pitted
3/4 cup blueberries
1 apple, cored and sliced

Process the fruit in a juicer or blender and serve.

Losing weight with a properly working digestion

The secret to losing weight permanently is having a properly working digestion, eating right and plenty of enzymes in your body. You can use Bio-Build and some simple weight loss exercises.

The main reason why people these days are overweight or have fat in unwanted places is because their digestion is not working properly. The body needs to be able to digest everything.

If your body cannot digest some of its food, then it stores the food for later use. Your body then starts to gain fat because of all the excess food waste that is being unnecessarily stored.

Eating large amounts of highly processed foods has this affect on many digestive systems, since most of the ingredients in many of today's processed food is mostly indigestible.

The best types of foods to eat are organic foods. If you are not able to get organic foods then you can still eat commercially grown foods on a daily basis but getting your digestion under control is a must if you want to lose weight and build a good-working, strong and healthy body.

The key is to get your digestion working to its full potential so that you absorb most of the fat and nutrients you need for your health. That way your body will be getting all it needs to be healthy without storing excess waste.

Amino acids and what they do

Amino acids are essential in a healthy digestion and in keeping your weight regulated. All enzymes are created by amino acids. Each enzyme uses between 100 to 1000 amino acids it its creation.

Once the enzyme is created, then your body uses it to break down a fat, a protein or a carbohydrate molecule. This is the way our bodies help to digest and use the energy.

Our body needs 22 amino acids to properly digest nutrients. We can only produce 10 of the 22 amino acids. The other 12 amino acids we get from our food. The main problem here is that if any of the food is cooked or processed in any way we lose all digestive enzymes in any food we consume.

The food may still have many good proteins, carbohydrates, fats and starches that will help our bodies grow, but we also need the digestive enzymes to properly digest everything.

Unlike fat and starch, the human body does not store excess amino acids for later use. The amino acids must be in the food everyday, otherwise we will not be able to use them.

Thus, if the food we eat is processed and does not contain any amino acids, our bodies have to try to get the amino acids from somewhere else

66

to properly digest the food. This can be the start of many problems including bad digestion.

BioBuild, an amino acid supplement, is an excellent way to have all your essential and non-essential amino acids that your body needs everyday. I personally use their product.

Having all the proper amino acids to digest everything that we put into our bodies is essential, if we want to stay healthy, slim and fit.

Some very simple weight loss exercises

The best weight loss exercise is doing something you love to do that makes you sweat. If you can find something to do that you like doing a lot and it's something that makes you break out into a sweat, then do that until you sweat! This will help greatly in reducing your weight and give your body a healthy shape.

There is swimming, biking, hiking, jogging and yoga that will do the trick as well, but don't over stress yourself. As soon as your body breaks out in a sweat, stop and rest. The sweat is an indication that your body is burning fat and needs to rest for regeneration.

Going on a daily walk is a very good weight loss exercise. You not only get fresh air and lots of things to look at but you also work your body to its limit of breaking a sweat. Walk with a big stride, stretching each leg. Walk as fast as you can. Quick, long strides help the body to reach its sweating point faster. It also builds great muscle.

Going to the gym is also a great way to lose weight. Lifting weights and doing strenuous exercises will help you to lose weight and at the same time help to build a strong and tough body. Remember, to never overstress yourself unless you are planning on becoming a body builder.

If you are or know someone that could benefit from losing weight, then look for

Digest Alive: Lose Weight and Build a Great Body Naturally

In this book, I give valuable information on how anyone can lose as much weight as they want and build a sexy, strong and healthy appearance. By balancing our three bodies, by eating right and by toning certain muscles in the body.

Reference directory

The American Dental Association (ADA)

Dr. Elena Koles, MD - Alternative medicine Chicago

Ron Harder, - A Nutritional health consultant

MayoClinic - Healthy digestion: Keeping on track

Rosemary Ann Ogilvie - All About Digestion

Alexis Black - Heartburn medications do more harm than good

Ron Kurtus - Heartburn Health Issue

Glossary of Terms

Chyme Chyme is the liquid substance found in the stomach before passing through to the small intestine.

Digestive enzymes Digestive enzymes are enzymes in the alimentary tract with a purpose of breaking down components of food so that they can be digested by the system.

Esophagus The esophagus (also spelled oesophagus or œsophagus), is a muscular tube through which food passes from the mouth area to the stomach.

Exocrine glands Exocrine glands are glands that secrete helpful digestive enzymes into ducts.

Gastrointestinal The gastrointestinal tract or GI tract, is also called the digestive tract. It is the system of organs which takes in food, digests it to extract energy and nutrients, and expels the remaining waste.

Heuristic churning Heuristic churning is a process in which the digestion mixes everything up inside the stomach for better absorption.

Hydrochloric acid The chemical compound hydrochloric acid is the (water-based) solution of hydrogen chloride gas (HCl) It is a strong acid, that is produced and used in your stomach to break down food into proteins and energy for the body.

LES Lower esophageal sphincter or LES is a muscle that is located at the very end of your esophagus. It opens to let chewed food into your stomach and closes to keep stomach acid out of your throat.

Lymphatic system The lymphatic system is a complex network of lymphoid organs, lymph nodes, lymph ducts, lymph tissues, lymph capillaries and lymph vessels that produce and transport lymph fluid from tissues to the circulatory system. The lymphatic system is a major component of the immune system.

Mucous membranes The mucous membranes are mostly involved in absorption and secretion. They line various body cavities that are exposed to the external environment and internal organs such as the skin, at the nostrils, the lips, the ears, the genital area, and the anus.

Peristalsis Peristalsis is the contraction of stomach muscles to propel contents through the digestive tract.

Phytochemicals Phytochemicals are naturally occurring chemicals from a plant source.

Polysaccharides Polysaccharides are

relatively complex carbohydrates.

Salivary glands The salivary glands are exocrine glands in the mouth that produce saliva.

Sialagogue Sialagogue Is an herb which stimulates the secretion of saliva from the salivary glands.

Xerostomia Xerostomia is the medical term for a dry mouth due to a lack of saliva.

Digest Alive Note pages

78